Just the
Right Dose

Your Smart Guide to
Prescription Drugs &
How to Take Them
Safely

Marijke Vroomen Durning, RN.

Just the Right Dose: Your Smart Guide to Prescription Drugs & How to Take Them Safely

By Marijke Vroomen Durning, RN

Reviewed by Rob Campbell, Reg. Pharmacist

Table of Contents

Just the Right Dose: Your Smart Guide to Prescription Drugs & How to Take Them Safely
by Marijke Vroomen Durning, RN

First Printing: 2015
ISBN - 978-0-9940300-0-9 (electronic)
ISBN - 978-0-9940300-1-6 (print)
Montreal, Quebec, Canada

Cover Image - iStock
Cover Design - Jasia Stuart
Content review: Rob Campbell, Reg. Pharmacist, University of Toronto, 1978
Copy editing - Hilda Brucker
Author Photo: Mark Bennington

In **Just the Right Dose: Your Smart Guide to Prescription Drugs & How to Take Them Safely,** you'll find answers to the most common questions about over-the-counter and prescription medications, as well as tips on topics such as:

- Understanding your prescription
- Why it's important to follow the directions,
- What types of pills you should never break or chew, and why
- The most common types of medicines (such as cream, suppositories, injections)
- Remembering to take your medications
- Swallowing that pill or capsule
- Getting rid of unused drugs
- And more!

Acknowledgements

Thank you to everyone who helped make this book possible, from my husband Peter, sons Kevin and Matthew, and daughter Anne, to my friends and colleagues who have encouraged me as I nurtured my writing career.

This book would not be possible without the help of Rob Campbell, who reviewed the information to ensure that it was correct and as up-to-date as possible, and Jasia Stuart, who designed the book's cover. It also would not have been possible to write this book without the thousands of patients I've cared for over the years. It was through this work that I learned about the gaps of health knowledge that exist and it was one of the driving forces when I began my career as a health writer. As I taught them, they taught me.

Thank you for purchasing *Just the Right Dose: Your Smart Guide to Prescription Drugs & How to Take Them Safely.* I hope that you will find the information useful and that I answer your questions about prescription drugs.

To let others know about the book, please take a few moments to spread the word by leaving a review of the book either on Amazon or at the site from which you bought it. These reviews help raise the profile of the book so others may find it more easily. It would also be a big help if you could spread the word on social media, by posting about it on Facebook, LinkedIn, Twitter, and Pinterest.

Thank you.

Introduction

Taking medicines is a daily ritual for many people. Others rarely fill a prescription or take an over-the-counter pain reliever. Whichever category you fall into, it's important to understand what drugs you're taking or giving to someone else. From what may seem like secret codes on prescriptions to what to do if you have side effects, there can be many questions.

Your pharmacist is your medication expert and the best person to ask about anything related to drugs, either prescription or over-the-counter. Medical doctors, nurse practitioners, dentists, and other healthcare professionals who can prescribe drugs know which medicines and doses to order for their patients. They know about side effects and other issues related to the medicines. But it is the pharmacists who are the most up-to-date on drugs and medicine information.

Pharmacists are also the gatekeepers for your drug records. It may be tempting and easier to stop at the closest drugstore after you've been to an urgent care clinic or your doctor's office, but it's important to try to only use one pharmacy for all your medicines. This keeps all your records in one place and the pharmacists can quickly find out who has ordered drugs for you. This helps lower the risk that you may take medicines that could work against each other.

Chapter 1: Understanding Your Prescription

It's an old joke that doctors have terrible handwriting and that no one can read what they write. Unfortunately, this is true sometimes. So, it's important that you understand what your doctor has written on your prescription. This is the first step to being an informed patient.

Tip

When you get a prescription, ask the person who wrote it to read it with you. Ask questions if anything is not clear.

Prescriptions are written in a type of shorthand that is standard across the medical community. A prescription written in one city or state/province should be understood in another. A prescription should always include:

- Name of the patient
- Date the prescription is written
- Name of the medicine
- Dose of the medicine
- Frequency (how often the medicine should be taken)

- Method of administration (by mouth, on the skin, suppository, etc.)
- Duration (how long the medicine should be taken)
- Number of refills allowed
- Prescriber's* signature and license number

A prescription that is missing any of the above information is not complete. **It should not be filled by a pharmacist.**

Although not absolutely necessary, it's helpful if the prescription mentions what the drugs are for - such as for pain, sleep, or anxiety.

Prescribers can be a medical doctor, nurse practitioner, dentist, podiatrist, and some other healthcare professionals.

Prescription specifics

Date of the prescription

CHAPTER 1: UNDERSTANDING YOUR PRESCRIPTION

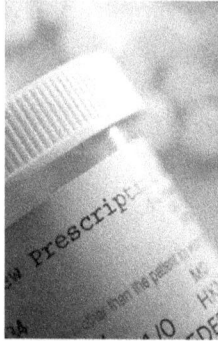

The date the prescription was written must be on the sheet and the prescription expires (is no longer valid) after one year from that date. Sometimes prescriptions are written for medicines that you don't need right away. You only take these medicines when you need them. Even though you may not need these drugs right away, the prescription still expires one year after the date it was ordered. This means the pharmacist can no longer fill it.

Tip

Bring your prescription to the drugstore as soon as you have it, even if you do not plan on taking the drug right away. It will be entered into your record to be used later, if and when you need it. It also

***means you don't have to look for the
prescription when you do need it.***

Medication name

The name of the drug written on the
prescription can be generic (the chemical
name) or the brand name. Many drug names
are very similar, such as Celexa and
Celebrex, so don't be shy to ask if you are not
sure of the drug's name.

Tip

***In most cases, generic drugs are as
good as a brand name drug, but cheaper.
However, this is not always the case and
your physician or nurse practitioner may
insist that you be given a brand name and
write "no substitutions" on your
prescription.***

Dose

Every prescription must say how much of the
medicine you should take. The amount can be
specific (5 mg., 2 tablespoons, 1 suppository)

or it can be a range ("one or two tablets" or "from 325 to 650 mg).

Tip

If you are taking liquid medicines, be sure to use a measuring tool (spoon or syringe) that is meant to be used for medicines. A regular spoon is not accurate enough for medicines nor is a measuring spoon meant for cooking.

Frequency

There are different ways a healthcare provider can write how often or how frequently you should take your medicine. Your doctor may want you to take the drug every four, six, eight, or 12 hours, for example. These precise instructions keep a steady level of medicine in your body. This helps the medication work properly.

Sometimes your prescription may say "three times a day," or "four times a day," instead of saying how many hours in between doses. In this case, it's best to keep the medication

doses as evenly spread out throughout the
day as possible, but there is a bit of leeway as
long as the medication is taken at fairly
equally spaced times.

If you're told to take a drug every six hours,
you may have to take it at 6 a.m., noon, 6
p.m. and midnight. However, if the
prescription says that you should take it four
times a day, you may be able to take it as
soon as you wake up (assuming you're not
sleeping in until noon!), around lunch time,
around supper time and then before you go to
bed.

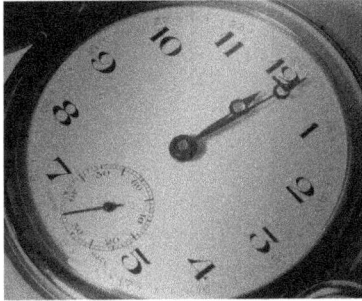

Your prescription may also say something like
"take before meals as needed," or "take every
four to six hours as needed." There should still

be a time frame to be sure you don't take them too often.

Of course, you should always check with your pharmacist for the best time schedule for your individual prescriptions.

Tip

Changing your clocks to and from Daylight Savings Time (DST) or traveling through time zones may throw a strict medication schedule off kilter. Ask your pharmacist how you should manage your medications with the extra hours or shortened days.

Method

Not all medicines are taken the same way. Most prescriptions are for pills, capsules, or liquids that you take by mouth. The shorthand abbreviation for medications you swallow is "po," for "per os." But there are also suppositories (vaginal and rectal), injections, eye or ear drops, creams, and more.

CHAPTER 1: UNDERSTANDING YOUR PRESCRIPTION

It's important that you understand how to take each specific drug. Some people have taken or given medications the wrong way. If this happens, the medical condition being treated might not get better and could get worse. It may seem obvious how a medicine should be taken, but sometimes the obvious is what can trip us up.

Keep in mind that there are some medications that may be regularly taken one way, but can also be used another way, depending on the problem it's treating. For example, the antibiotic vancomycin is usually given intravenously, or IV. But, it may be ordered to be taken by mouth to treat certain illnesses. Always be sure you know how you are to take your medications.

Duration and refills (repeats)

Your prescription should say how long you need to take your medicine, unless you have to take it over a long period of time or indefinitely. A prescription for antibiotics may say "x 10 days." This means you need to take the drug for 10 days. If your prescription is for a longer time or goes indefinitely, the prescription should tell the pharmacist how many times the order can be refilled before you need to get a new prescription.

Tip

Even if you are feeling better before your prescription is finished, it's important that you finish all the medicine, especially for drugs like antibiotics. Feeling better is not the same thing as eliminating the problem altogether.

Signature and license number

A prescription is not valid if it's not signed by the prescribing physician, nurse practitioner, or other healthcare provider. The signature must also have his or her license number for the state or province.

Chapter 2: Filling Your Prescription

Once you have brought your prescription to the drugstore, or it has been called in or faxed by the medical or dental office, the information will be added to your record. If you don't have a file at the drugstore, the technician or pharmacist will ask you several questions to set up your file. They will ask for your birth date, whether you take any other medicines (prescription and over-the-counter), if you have any allergies, and your insurance information.

When you get your medicine, especially if it's the first time you are taking it, you should ask your pharmacist to go over the prescription with you. You want to make sure you know:

- The drugs you received are the ones that were prescribed
- How much you should take, how often, and for how long
- If there are any warnings, such as take the medicine on an empty stomach or with food, avoiding certain types of food or, staying out of the sun
- How the medicine should be stored (room temperature, in the fridge, in a

dark place)
- If this medicine has potential interactions with the ones you already take (including over-the-counter drugs or supplements)
- Why you are taking it
- If you should stop other medicines while you are taking this one
- When you should start noticing that the medicine is working
- Whether there are side effects you should be aware of
- What to do if you miss a dose
- When you should contact the person who wrote the prescription if there are side effects or it seems like the medicine is not working

Tip

Ask your pharmacist for a print out of all your medicines and keep this in your wallet or purse. If you need to see a doctor or there is an emergency, you can give this list to the medical staff instead of having to remember what you are taking. This list is also very helpful if you are traveling, especially to another country.

Once you bring your medicine home, it's a good idea to count the pills to make sure you've been given the right number. Pharmacists and their technicians are human and sometimes they do make mistakes. Look closely at the medications. Get to know what they look like. Many drugs look similar to others, so look at the shape, and color, and note if there are any markings on them.

Tip

Some people place one of each pill on a white piece of paper with the name of the medicine below. They then take a photo with a digital camera or smart phone, to help remember what the pills look like.

Never put your pills in another pill bottle. Unless you are using a daily pill reminder container, drugs should always stay in their original containers. This is for safety and can help prevent accidental overdoses or mistaken doses.

Tip

If you are filling a weekly pill container

(called a dosette in Canada and the UK) for someone else, leave a list of the medicines and the times they should be taken in case someone else becomes involved. Weekly pill boxes should have names of the medicines attached to it. Some pharmacies will do this for you.

Chapter 3: Taking Your Meds (Or Giving Them To Someone In Your Care)

Medications come in many forms. Some can only be given one way, while others may be given in different ways. The most common form of medication is oral, by mouth - tablets, capsules, and liquids.

Some people find it hard to swallow pills or capsules, especially the bigger ones. If this happens to you, it may be tempting to break a pill in half or open a capsule to pour the contents onto a spoon of jam or peanut butter, but **you should only do this if the pharmacist has said you can**.

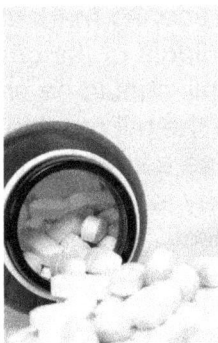

CHAPTER 3: TAKING YOUR MEDS (OR GIVING THEM TO SOMEONE IN YOUR CARE)

Not all pills should be broken or chewed, and not all capsules should be opened. Many have a special coating that releases the drug when it has reached a certain part of your stomach or colon. Others have a gradual drug release system, where some of the medicine is released as soon as you take it, and the rest comes out bit by bit over the next few hours. If you break these pills or open the capsules, you could end up overdosing, causing serious side effects or even death.

If your pharmacist has said that you can break the pill to either make it easier to swallow or because you are taking half the usual dose, there should be a scoring mark or a groove (line) across the middle of the tablet. This marks where the pill should be broken. You may want to snap the pill or tablet in half with your hands or touse a knife to cut it, but the best and safest way is to use a pill cutter. Pill cutters are specifically designed for this purpose. Pill cutters can be found at any drugstore.

Tips

CHAPTER 3: TAKING YOUR MEDS (OR GIVING THEM TO SOMEONE IN YOUR CARE)

A new, sharp paint scraper blade, used only to cut pills, is another option to help cut scored pills.

The blades in the pill cutters get dull after a while. The more you use the cutter, the more quickly this will happen. If you notice any crumbling from the pills or you start having difficulty cutting them, replace the cutter as soon as possible.

One danger of breaking a pill by hand or using a kitchen knife is that one side of the pill may end up being larger than the other. This can cause uneven dosing if you only need to take half the dose. It may not seem obvious to you that one side is slightly smaller than the other, but it can be important with some medications. Breaking the pill by hand or with a knife can also make part of the pill crumble. Even if you take both halves of the pill - you're just cutting them to make them easier to swallow - you may not get the full dose since some of the crumbs have been lost when the pill was broken.

Finally, don't split pills ahead of time if you can avoid it. The pill's coating helps keep the pill's strength. If the coating is lost or broken, the medication can break down over time as it is exposed to oxygen and moisture.

If you are crushing pills, there are pill crushers also available at the drug store. Using two spoons to crush a pill can cause little bits of the pill to get lost in the process. A pill crusher keeps everything in one place, so you get the full dose.

Tip

Be sure to clean out the pill crusher after every use. Leaving behind crumbs can add extra medicine to the following doses.

Swallowing a pill or capsule

Swallowing something whole goes against our nature. Your gag reflex usually keeps this from happening, so it's not unusual for people to have trouble swallowing pills, no matter how tiny they are. Here are some tricks that may help you if this is a problem:

When possible, sit or stand up while taking your medicine. Sitting straight up or standing gives the medicine a straight path down.

Don't stretch your neck. If you watch people taking pills, you'll see that some look up at the ceiling. This stretches their neck. If you've tried this and it doesn't work, try doing the opposite, and look down before swallowing. This relaxes the muscles around your neck, giving the pill more room to slide down. This is helpful for taking capsules, which don't have the weight of a tablet.

Place the pill on the back of your tongue. By placing the pill on the back of your tongue, as soon as you take a sip of liquid, it should push the medicine back and down your throat.

Place the pill on the tip of your tongue. Some people find that if they have the pill at the very front of their mouth and then they take a big sip of their drink, the pill will move along with the liquid.

Sip first. Take a sip or gulp of liquid first to wet your mouth, then try taking the pill.

Use a straw. Some people find that the suction that happens when you use a straw helps them swallow the pill.

Take a deep breath. Place the pill in your mouth, take a deep breath, and then drink.

Crush the pill if you may. If your pharmacist has said you can crush your pill or open the capsule, do so and mix it with a favorite food, like apple sauce, peanut butter, or ice cream.

Ask for a liquid. If you truly can't swallow your pills, ask if there is a liquid alternative. Many medications are available in a liquid form that is meant for younger children who are not yet able to swallow pills.

Tip

If you have to take medications on a

regular basis and have trouble swallowing them, practice on mini candies or ask your pharmacist for empty capsules. Mini candies, like TicTacs are the perfect size to practice swallowing pills.

Sublingual medicines (under the tongue)

Some medicines must be taken by putting them under your tongue, where the drug is absorbed. This method is very fast acting and is used for drugs like nitroglycerin, which is given for angina (heart pain).

It is very easy to take medication this way, but there are a few things to keep in mind to make sure the medicine works as it should:

Take your oral medications first. If you take pills, capsules, or liquid medicines at the same time that your sublingual drug is due, take the ones you have to swallow first.

Don't smoke before taking your dose. Smoking constricts (tightens) your blood vessels, so it may affect how your sublingual medicine is absorbed. If you do smoke, try not to smoke for at least an hour before taking a sublingual medicine.

Place the pill under your tongue. Hold your head normally, allowing your tongue to hold the pill in place. It should dissolve quickly.

Wait before drinking or rinsing your mouth. Wait at least five minutes after taking your medicine before having a drink or rinsing your mouth, to be sure the drug has been completely absorbed.

Topical medicines (on the skin)

Some medications are applied directly to the skin. These include patches, creams, ointments, and gels. Some of these medicines are absorbed through the skin to get into your body, and some topical drugs target only the specific spot that the medicine touches.

Patches

CHAPTER 3: TAKING YOUR MEDS (OR GIVING THEM TO SOMEONE IN YOUR CARE)

Many medicines can be given by patch. For example, some help you manage pain and others may help you quit smoking. The advantage to medicines delivered through patches is that the dose usually lasts longer, and you don't have to swallow pills or take injections. The disadvantage is that if the patches aren't applied properly, you might not get the proper doses.

Check with your pharmacist about where you should put the patch. Not all parts of your body are equally good at absorbing drugs. Some medicines should be placed on the upper body, while others are placed behind the ear, for example.

Do not cut or divide your patch. If you think your dose is too high, don't cut or adjust the patch in any way without checking with your pharmacist.

Your skin should be clean and free of any oils or creams. If you've just had a shower or bath, dry your skin gently and wait a few minutes before applying the patch. The skin needs to be completely free of any type of oil or cream so the patch can stick and the medication can be absorbed properly.

Remove the old patch. This may sound obvious, but sometimes people forget to remove the old patch after putting on the new patch. Be sure to remove the old patch to so you don't get more of the drug than you should. Dispose the patch as instructed by your pharmacist.

Creams and ointments

You may receive a prescription for medicine in a cream or ointment form. As with the patches, it is important to make sure your skin is clean, dry, and free of any oils or other creams before applying the medicinal cream.

Before applying the cream, it's important to know:

- Where it should be applied
- How thickly the cream or ointment should be applied
- What to do if you get the cream or ointment outside of the area where it

should be applied
- Be sure to wash your hands after applying the medicine

Tip

Beware that some creams and ointments are dangerous for people who should not use them, such as testosterone cream, which may be prescribed for men. Women and children should not touch the cream, nor should they touch the skin where this cream has been applied, or towels or cloths that have touched the cream.

Inhaled medications

Medicine sometimes needs to go straight into the lungs. These are delivered by an inhaler - a device that lets you breathe in the drug. Inhalers comes in three types of devices:

- Metered-dose inhaler (MDI), which uses a chemical to push the medicine

    out of a cannister
- Dry powder inhaler
- Spinhaler
  (http://aerosol.ees.ufl.edu/healthaeroso
  l/section04-1b.html)

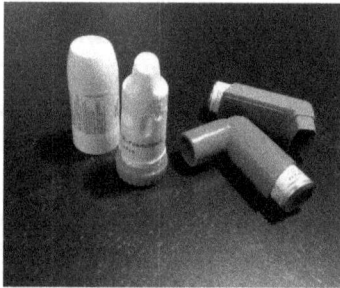

There is one other method that delivers inhaled medicine: a *nebulizer*. A nebulizer is a machine that turns medicine into a fine mist that you breathe in, using a facemask or mouthpiece. This is used most often in a hospital setting, but some people do have nebulizers at home. If you are going to use a nebulizer, be sure to read and follow the manufacturer's instructions so the medicine is delivered properly.

Inhaled medicines are usually used to treat

CHAPTER 3: TAKING YOUR MEDS (OR GIVING THEM TO SOMEONE IN YOUR CARE)

illnesses and conditions like asthma and chronic obstructive pulmonary disease (COPD). There are fast-acting "rescue" drugs and maintenance drugs. Rescue medicines are drugs that you take only as needed, for immediate relief of your symptoms. Maintenance medicines are taken regularly to prevent symptoms from happening in the first place. Some medications combine both rescue and maintenance drugs.

If you have an inhaler, be sure you understand the proper way to use it, so you get the drug's full dose. Your pharmacist should be able to answer questions about the device and how to make sure you've properly received the medicine.

Tip

If you have to take more than one puff from your inhaler or you have more than one kind of inhaled medicine to take, ask your pharmacist how much time you need to leave between puffs and which inhaler to use first.

Using a metered-dose inhaler

- ***Shake the inhaler*** to mix the medicine and remove the cap.
- ***Breathe out***, so your lungs are empty.
- ***Either put the inhaler to your lips or keep it an inch or so away,*** depending on what you were taught by your healthcare provider or pharmacist.
- ***Slowly start to breathe in*** and - at the same time - press down fully on the canister one time, all while breathing in the spray.
- **Try to hold your breath** for at least 10 seconds.

If you need a second puff or you're using a second type of inhaled medication, repeat the process.

If your medicine is a steroid, rinse your mouth with water or brush your teeth when finished your final dose.

To use a powder inhaler or spinhaler, follow

the manufacturer's instructions. *If you are
using a dry powder inhaler, do not turn it
upside down once you have activated the
dose because you will lose some of the
powder and receive too small of a dose.*

Tip

**If you find it's hard to get the timing
right with a metered-dose inhaler
(breathing out, pressing the canister, and
then breathing in the medicine) or you're
giving the medication to a child or adult
who can't help, ask your healthcare
provider or pharmacist about using a
spacer. A spacer is a plastic tube
(canister) that sits between the inhaler and
your mouth. Or, you could ask if you can
have a medicine that is delivered with a
dry powder instead.**

**To use a spacer, prepare the inhaler as
usual and then insert the mouthpiece into
one end of the spacer. Place the other end
of the spacer either in your mouth (if it has
a mouthpiece) or over your nose and**

mouth (if it has a mask). Breathe in deeply five or six times to be sure you have breathed in all the medication.

Using dry powder or spinhalers

These devices can be quite different, depending on the manufacturer. To be sure you are using your device properly, ask your pharmacist for a demonstration and check the instructions.

Eye drops, ointments, or gels

Eye drops, ointments, or gels are prescribed or recommended for many reasons. Some people need them to keep their eyes from getting too dry, others need them to treat serious conditions like glaucoma. As with any other medicine, eye drops, ointments, and gels should be used as directed.

Drops

- *Wash your hands.*
- *Check the bottle* to make sure the fluid

(if you can see it) is clear and doesn't have anything in it.

- *Take off the cap* but be sure not to touch the tip of the bottle with your fingers, your eye, or eyelid.
- *Tilt your head back.*
- *Gently pull down on the skin just below your eye,* making a sort of pocket. Look up.
- *Hold the bottle with your right hand* if you're right handed, your left hand if left handed, with the nozzle or tip pointing down. Bring it as close to your eye as you can without actually touching it to your eye.
- *Squeeze the bottle* so that one drop (or more, depending on the prescription), drips into the pocket.
- *Close your eye for a minute or so*. Also, pinch the bridge of your nose for a minute to 90 seconds.
- *Recap the bottle* and wash your hands.

Ointments or gels

- *Wash your hands.*

- ***Take off the cap,*** but be sure not to touch the open tip of the bottle with your fingers, your eye, or eyelid.
- ***Tilt your head back.***
- ***Pull down gently on the skin below your eye***, making a pocket of sorts. Look up.
- ***Squeeze the tube*** to allow a small ribbon of the product to come out into the pocket.
- ***Close your eye for a few seconds.***
- ***Recap the tube.*** If any ointment or gel is left on the nozzle, wipe it off with a clean tissue to keep the medicine from gumming up the opening.
- ***Wash your hands.***

Tip

If you are using drops or ointments for your eyes, you may find that one or both eyes are "glued" shut when you wake up in the morning or after you've taken a nap. If this happens, use a clean cloth with warm water to gently wipe your eye, from the outside to the inside, toward your nose.

Ear drops

- ***Check to see if the fluid in the bottle*** looks as it should, as recommended with the eye drops.
- ***Shake the bottle*** for a few seconds to mix the fluid, if instructed.
- *Since cold liquid can feel uncomfortable in your ear, you may want to hold the bottle in your hand for a minute or so, to warm it up a bit.*
- ***Withdraw the medication in the dropper*** (if the bottle doesn't have a direct drip at the top).
- ***Tilt your head to the opposite side*** (if you are putting the drops in the right ear, tilt your head sideways to the left).
- ***Hold the top of your ear between your thumb and index (pointing) finger,*** and pull gently back and upward. This will open your ear canal. If you are giving ear drops to a young child, pull the ear back and downward for the same effect.
- ***Drop in the prescribed or***

recommended number of drops. If you are giving the ear drops to someone else, hold the bottle so that a drop appears at the opening - then allow it to run down the side of the ear canal, instead of dropping them straight in the ear. This is especially helpful if you are giving the drops to a child who had an ear infection. It keeps the drops from hitting the eardrum, which will cause pain.

- ***Keep the tilted position*** for a few minutes.
- ***Insert a cotton swab into the canal*** (not deeply) if your healthcare provider has told you to do so.

Tip

Some drops need "pumping" for children who have tubes in their ears. If your child has ear tubes, ask your pharmacist if you must do this. The drops are placed in the ear canal and then you "close" the ear with the skin flap. Gently pump about five times to push the drops down.

Nasal sprays

Nasal sprays deliver medication directly to the nasal passages.

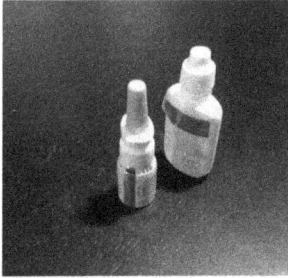

To administer a spray:

- ***Blow your nose gently if you can***. Blowing too hard can close up the sinuses.
- ***Keep your head slightly forward***, about 20 degrees.
- ***Insert the tip*** of the bottle just inside the nostril.
- ***Block the other nostril*** with your index (pointing) finger of the other hand.
- ***Squeeze the bottle or activate the***

trigger and breathe in deeply at the same time. Hold your breath for 10 seconds and then breathe out through your mouth - not the nose.

Repeat on the other side as directed or if necessary.

Nasal drops

- **Prepare as for the spray.**
- **Lie down** with your face up to the ceiling.
- **Do not allow the tip of the dropper to touch your nose.**
- **Drop in the prescribed or recommended number of drops.**
- **Sit up and bend your head forward a bit.** Stay this way for a minute or two.

Suppositories

Suppositories can be given in the rectum or vagina. Rectal suppositories are prescribed either because the patient cannot tolerate swallowing medication or because the medication needs to be delivered directly to that area. Vaginal suppositories deliver medicine directly to the vaginal area.

Store your suppositories as directed. Many suppositories should be kept in a cool dark place so they keep their shape. This makes them easier to insert. If you are not sure about your prescription, ask your pharmacist. Suppositories that don't need to be kept cold may become soft with handling. Ask your pharmacist if you can put the medication in the fridge for about 30 minutes before administering it if you find this to be a problem.

- *Try to empty your bowels before inserting rectal suppositories,* unless the suppository is being taken for constipation. This may help reduce the need to go to the bathroom after you have put in the suppository.
- *Squat if possible,* or rest on your side, bending the leg on top and keeping the other leg straight.
- *Remove the suppository from the*

> ***package/foil.***
> - ***If needed, you could moisten the tip***
>   of the suppository with water.
> - ***Push the suppository into the***
>   ***rectum or vagina*** far enough that it
>   doesn't come right back out.
> - ***Wash your hands.***
> - ***Try to sit or lie still for a few minutes***,
>   and hold in the suppository as long as
>   possible.

Injections

Many people have to give themselves
injections (shots) or give them to someone
they are caring for.

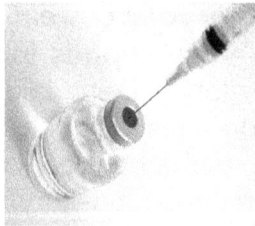

There are two types of injections that
someone may need to self-administer.
Subcutaneous injections, abbreviated as "sc"

or "sq," are given in the fatty tissue, just under
the skin. Intramuscular injections, abbreviated
as IM, are given directly into muscle.
Subcutaneous needles are shorter than IM
needles. Anyone who must take or give
injections should receive personal instruction
from a healthcare professional. The
information in this book is intended to serve
solely as a reminder for information that you
have already received.

Wash your hands. Always be sure that you
wash your hands before preparing and giving
an injection. The area you are in should also
be as clean as possible, to avoid
contamination. This is especially important if
you are away from home and may need to
give the injection in a public place.

Prepare your injection as directed. If you
have any questions about medication
preparation or how to store the drug, ask your
pharmacist. Here are some reminders for the
usual procedure:

- **Check the label** to be sure it is the
  correct medicine, particularly if the

prescription has just been filled or
refilled.
- **Inspect the contents** of the syringe or
vial for anything that does not appear
normal, such as anything floating in the
liquid, cloudiness if it should be clear,
etc.
- *Check the seal* on the container to be
sure that it is still properly sealed.
- *If you have a pen-delivery system, skip
the following steps and use your pen as
your healthcare provider taught you
and according to the manufacturer's
instructions.*
- **Wipe the top of the vial** with a piece of
gauze soaked with rubbing alcohol or
an alcohol swab. Be careful not to
touch the top once you've cleaned it. If
you do touch it, wipe it with alcohol
again.
- *Attach the needle to the syringe,* if it
is not already there.
- *Pull back the plunger on syringe*,
filling it with air to the amount of fluid
you will be taking out of the vial. For
example, if you have to take out 2 cc or
ml of medicine from the vial, you will

draw back the plunger on the syringe to
fill it with 2 ccs or mls of air. Be careful
to only hold the rounded bottom part of
the plunger, not the "stick" part, to keep
it sterile.

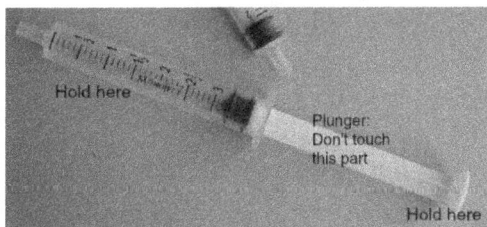

- *Remove the cap from the needle.* Be
  sure to keep it within easy reach.
- *Without touching the needle against
  anything else, push the needle
  through the rubber stopper* on the
  vial. Keep the needle at a 90-degree
  angle (straight in).
- *Once the needle is in,* turn the vial
  upside down, with the needle still
  inside.
- *Push the plunger slowly* to push the
  air from the syringe to the vial. Hold the
  needle in. Do not take it out.
- *Look in the vial* to be sure that the tip

of the needle is in the fluid, not poking
out above it into the air. Slowly begin to
pull back the plunger to take out the
right amount of medicine. Keep
checking to be sure that the tip of the
needle remains in the fluid in the vial.

- ***Keeping the syringe still upright,*** flick
the syringe with your finger or a pen to
push any air bubbles up to the top of
the syringe. Using the plunger, push the
air bubbles out of the syringe back up
into the bottle. Then pull back a bit on
the plunger again to fill that space with
medication, if you need to.
- ***Pull the needle out of the vial,*** making
sure that you don't touch the needle
against your hand or any objects.
- ***Carefully replace the cap,*** making
sure you don't touch the needle. If you
do touch the needle by accident,
replace it with a clean one before giving
the injection.

Giving the injection

- ***Check the skin in the spot where you will give the injection.*** Unless your physician, nurse, or pharmacist has told you otherwise, shots should not be given in areas where skin is damaged, reddened, or swollen.
- ***Don't use the same site each time.*** For some medicines, it's important that you use different parts of your body, rotating injection sites, so you're not always giving shots in the same place. A few medicines should be given in the same area. If you are not sure, ask your healthcare provider for instructions.
- ***Clean the skin.*** Using rubbing alcohol, clean the area where you'll be giving the injection. Let the alcohol dry naturally.
- ***Keep a clean swab with rubbing alcohol within easy reach.*** This is to use after you have given the injection.
- **Take the cap off the needle,** being careful not to touch the needle while doing so. If you do touch the needle, change it.

Subcutaneous injection

- ***Hold the syringe as if you are
  holding a dart*** with your right hand if
  you're right-handed, your left hand if
  you're left-handed. Use your other hand
  to take some skin between your thumb
  and index (pointing) finger, with a
  pinching motion.
- ***Using a 90-degree angle (straight in),***
  firmly but gently insert the needle into
  the skin. Don't force the needle or go
  too slowly.* When the injection
  technique is demonstrated to you by
  your healthcare professional, pay
  attention to how her wrist moves. This
  will demonstrate the right motion and
  force for the needle to penetrate the
  skin.
- ***Once the needle is in, slowly and
  steadily push the plunger*** with your
  thumb to inject the medicine.
- ***When all the medicine has gone in,***
  pull the needle straight out in one quick
  motion.
- ***Place the clean gauze over the***

injection site and press lightly. Your healthcare provider may have told you to rub the area after the shot. Otherwise, don't rub it.

- *Discard your used needle and syringe* in a proper container as you've been instructed to. Do not reuse your needles. They become duller each time they are used and reusing them may also lead to serious infections.

* The 90-degree rule is for most people, but there are exceptions. For some people, especially those with little fat, the needle may have to go in at a sharper angle. If you are not sure, please ask your healthcare professional.

Intramuscular injection

- *Hold the syringe as if you are holding a dart* with your right hand if you're right-handed, your left hand if you're left-handed.
- *Spread the skin flat* between your thumb and index finger with your other hand.

CHAPTER 3: TAKING YOUR MEDS (OR GIVING THEM TO SOMEONE IN YOUR CARE)

- ***Using a 90-degree angle, firmly and quickly insert the needle*** through the skin and into the muscle. Do not force the needle or go too slowly. When the injection technique is demonstrated to you by your healthcare professional, pay attention to how her wrist moves. This will demonstrate the right motion and force for the needle to penetrate the skin.
- *(This step may or may not be recommended by your healthcare professional. If you are not sure, please check with him or her for specific instructions: Place one hand on the syringe to hold it steady and use your other hand to pull back very slightly on the plunger. This is to check for blood. If blood comes up into the syringe, withdraw the needle without injecting the medicine, and discard it in the sharps container. Put gentle pressure on the injection site and prepare another injection for a new site.)*
- ***If you are not checking for blood or if you have checked and there is no blood,*** use firm pressure to press on

the plunger to inject the medication.

- *Once all the medicine is in,* pull out
  the needle straight out, using a quick
  motion.
- *Press an alcohol swab on the site*
  and hold there for about 30 seconds.
- *Dispose of your used needle and
  syringe* in a proper container as per
  your pharmacist's instructions. Do not
  reuse your needles. They become
  duller each time they are used and
  reusing them may also lead to serious
  infections.

Chapter 4 - Taking the medications

With Food, Without Food, Avoiding Certain Food Products

Medicines may come with instructions to take them on an empty stomach, to take them with food, or to avoid certain types of food while you are taking them. These instructions help make the drugs more effective, keep them from not working properly, and reduce the risk of bad side effects.

Take with food

There are a few reasons why some medicines should be taken with food:

- The drug may be better absorbed into the body with food
- Food may buffer the stomach from the medicine, preventing nausea or heartburn
- The food helps the body process the medication or ingredients in the medicine

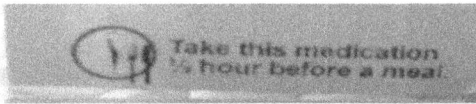

Take this medication ½ hour before a meal.

Take one hour before meals or two hours after

Some medicines should be taken on an empty stomach because food may stop the body from absorbing the medication properly. Instructions can range from 30 minutes before meals to a few hours after.

Do not take with dairy products

Dairy products can block the absorption of some types of medicines by binding the drug.

Do not consume grapefruit or grapefruit juice while taking this medication

Grapefruit and grapefruit juice can interfere with certain medications, such as some cholesterol-lowering drugs, sometimes making them much stronger than they should be. This doesn't happen all the time and it is unpredictable.

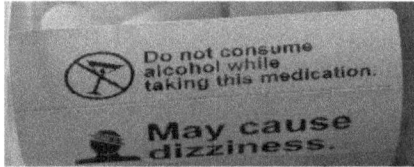

Avoid alcohol

Mixing alcohol with some medicines can cause severe side effects. Alcohol can also cause some medications not to work as well as they should. Some drugs can increase the alcohol's effect, making one drink feel like several.

Remembering to take your medications

Medicines work best when taken regularly, as prescribed. But, there are many reasons why some people find it hard to remember to take (or give) medications.

Here are some tips that might make it easier to remember:

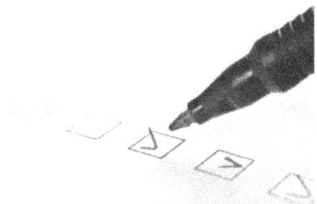

Write out a paper schedule. If you're taking medicine for a short period of time, such as antibiotics for 7 days, make a schedule. Put the schedule in an obvious place, like on your fridge door. List the doses (example: morning, afternoon, night) and the days. Cross off each dose as you take it.

Put a label on the bottle if you are giving (or taking yourself) a liquid medicine, with the same kind of schedule list. You can cross off the doses as you take or give them.

Make an electronic schedule. Instead of using paper to mark off your doses, do it on your computer, tablet, or smartphone.

Leave medicine in an obvious place. If it is safe to do so, leave morning or night medicines next to your toothbrush or grooming supplies, or on your bedside table. If your medicine is to be taken with breakfast, place it (or something that will remind you to take it) beside your breakfast bowl or mug. *If you have children visiting, please remember to put all drugs out of reach while they are around.*

Plan ahead. Use a weekly/daily pill box, refilled once a week. Some pharmacists can offer this service.

Set alarms. Set your smartphone to remind you by text or alarm to take your medicine. If you don't have a smartphone, an alarm clock or a watch with an alarm function would work too.

Did you forget to take your medicine?

Ask your healthcare provider what you should do if you forget to take a dose. For some medications, you may be told to take it as soon as you remember, as long as it's not too close to your next dose. Do not double up your medications unless you are specifically told to do so.

Time changes

If you travel and change time zones or have to reset your clocks because of changes to and from Daylight Savings Time, you may have to change how you take your medications.

In some situations, a change of an hour or two may not make a difference in your medicine schedule, but check with your healthcare provider or pharmacist to be sure. You may be told to push your scheduled dose back or ahead by a half hour one day before the time change and then, the following next day, to take it at the (new) regular time. This prevents an extra long gap between doses.

More drastic time changes will certainly affect how you should adapt your schedule. Your pharmacist can help you with a plan that is best for you.

Adverse Effects/Events

All drugs can cause side effects. Side effects

are usually unwanted or undesirable. The medical community calls them adverse effects or adverse events.

There are many possible side effects.

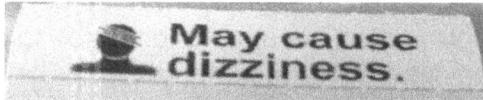

Some of the most common side effects include:

- Nausea
- Diarrhea
- Constipation
- Drowsiness
- Stimulation (feeling "hyper")
- Dizziness
- Lightheadedness
- Dry mouth

Changes in mental status can also happen when someone starts to take a new drug, particularly among older people. If someone you know is showing signs of a sudden personality change or seems to be more confused or disoriented than usual, check with the pharmacist to see if this could be caused by the new medication.

Other side effects may be caused by something that reacts with the medicine. For example, some medications cause *photosensitivity*. Your sensitivity to the sun, or photosensitivity, can get worse while you take the drug. When you pick up your prescription, it should have a warning label on it to tell you to stay out of the sun if the drug can cause photosensitivity.

When you read the list of side effects that a drug can cause, it's important to remember that the drug's manufacturer must list all side effects that have been reported, no matter how rare. This is why these side effect lists can be very long and sound scary.

If you notice any side effects from your medicine, you should report them to your healthcare provider. If the problems are mild, your pharmacist might be able to give you some tips to lessen the side effect. If you have any serious side effects or you are concerned, contact your healthcare provider as soon as possible.

Please remember that unless your healthcare provider has told you otherwise, do not stop taking your medication because of side effects. Stopping some medications suddenly, or discontinuing a medicine that is causing side effects without replacing it with something else, could cause more problems.

Throwing Out Unused Medications

Many people have unused or unfinished medicines, or over-the-counter products that have expired, in their homes. It may be tempting to throw these drugs in the trash, in the toilet, or down the drain. Please don't. This is not a safe practice because the drugs may affect the environment.

Ask your pharmacist what you should do about returning unwanted or unused medications. Many drug stores will collect and dispose of them.

Abuse of prescription medicines

Abuse of prescription medicines has always

been a problem for some people, but the problem seems to be growing, given the ever increasing number of drugs now available.

According to the <u>National Institutes of Health (NIH)</u> (http://www.drugabuse.gov/drugs-abuse/commonly-abused-drugs-charts/commonly-abused-prescription-drugs-chart) in the United States, the most commonly abused prescription drugs are:

- Depressants
- Opioids and morphine-related pain medications
- Stimulants

Depressant medicines include sleeping pills and anti-anxiety medicines, such as *benzodiazepines* and barbiturates. These drugs can be and often are life-savers for people who need them, but they can also be abused by people who want to feel the effects that the medications may provide, such as intense happiness and excitement (*euphoria*) and lowered inhibitions.

Opioids and morphine-related medicines are most often given to reduce or manage pain. They can also bring on a feeling of euphoria when taken by someone who does not have pain.

Stimulants, such as *amphetamines* and *methylphenidate*, are frequently abused by people seeking the feeling of increased energy and excitement. These drugs are legitimately used by people with attention deficit hyperactive disorder (ADHD).

Tolerance, physical dependence, and addiction

We often hear the words tolerance, physical dependence, and addiction related to drugs, and it's easy to confuse them.

In 2001, the American Academy of Pain Medicine, the American Pain Society, and the American Society of Addiction Medicine published definitions of tolerance, physical dependence, and addiction.

They wrote that with *tolerance*, you are in a state of adaptation. Your body has adapted to the drug and it no longer works as well at the dose you've been taking. If you are taking pain medications, your body can become used to the regular dose. After a while, that regular dose may not act as well and you need a stronger dose to do the same thing.

Physical dependence is a state of adaptation that gives you withdrawal symptoms if you suddenly stop taking the drug or you suddenly lower the dose.

Finally, *addiction* is more psychological than physical. The organizations said that people who are addicted to a drug show compulsive, uncontrollable use of the drug, they crave the drug, and they continue to use it despite harm that it causes.

In other words, with addiction, there is drug-seeking behavior and the user will continue to use the drug, even knowing that his behavior can cause harm to himself or others. With physical dependence, there is a physical feeling of being uncomfortable when you no longer have the drug.

Chapter 5 - Odds and Ends

Generic versus brand names

When researchers are working on a new medication, it is given a *generic* or general name, such as acetaminophen, dimenhydrinate, and sildenafil. These three drugs are now commonly known by brand names such as: Tylenol®, Dramamine® (Gravol® in Canada), and Viagra®. Brand names are the names that companies give their specific version of a generic drug.

As a rule, when a new medicine can be sold, the company that developed the drug has a patent (license) for several decades. This company is the only one that can produce and sell that drug for a set time. Once the patent expires, other companies may make and sell the medicine under their own name. These versions are usually cheaper than the original formula.

As a rule, all formulations (products made from the formula) are made with the same medicinal ingredients - the parts that make up the active medicine part of the drug. But each manufacturer may use different non-medicinal (inactive) ingredients to finish the product.

Non-medicinal ingredients may hold together medicinal ingredients or give the drug its color or taste. For this reason, not all generics are 100% alike. They should all work the same way and be as effective as each other. And most often they are. But there are cases where the non-medicinal ingredients in one generic version may slightly change how the drug works or they may cause a different side effect.

When you get a prescription, it may be written with either name - the generic or the brand name. In some situations, your healthcare provider may not want you to take the generic drug and she will write on the prescription "no substitutions." This means the pharmacist must give the original brand name medicine and not a generic. In some areas, the "no substitution" message must be handwritten or, if it's printed on the prescription sheet, it must be initialed by the prescriber.

If the person who wrote the prescription does not mention that the drug must be a brand name, you may ask the pharmacist if there is a generic equivalent. The pharmacist may already be in the habit of giving generic drugs when filling prescriptions.

Keep in mind that your insurance plan might not pay for the cost difference between the brand name drug and the generic option. Generic drugs can be up to 70% cheaper than their brand name equivalents, so ask your doctor or pharmacist for details.

Over-the-counter, behind-the-counter, and prescription medicines

Why are some drugs kept on the drugstore shelves, while others are behind the counter and you must ask for them? Why are other medicines only available if a healthcare provider says you may take them?

All medications have the potential to cause serious harm, even death. For this reason, it's important to understand that even over-the-counter medications that you can buy straight off a shelf, have guidelines about who should take them, who should not take them, how they should be taken, and how often.

Over-the-counter (OTC) medicines

Over-the-counter medicines can be bought from drugstores, and many grocery, general, and convenience stores, as well as online. You don't need a prescription to buy them. The most common OTC drugs are for pain, fever, constipation, diarrhea, cold and flu symptoms, or allergies.

If you're already taking medicines for other reasons, please check with your pharmacist before taking any OTC products, including eye drops and nose sprays. There are some drugs that should never be taken together, or should be taken with caution.

If you plan on taking more than one type of OTC drug, you should read the ingredients of each product closely. It's possible that two (or more) medicines have some of the same ingredients. If you take both, you may be taking double the recommended dose. For example, many cold medicines contain acetaminophen, but so do some pills for headaches. These could cause serious harm if taken together.

There are also some medicines that you must not take if you have certain illnesses or conditions, such as high blood pressure or glaucoma (high pressure in your eye). The medicine labels should have these warnings, but check with your pharmacist if you are not sure.

Over-the-counter medicines are not meant to be taken for long periods of time unless your healthcare provider has told you to do so. If you need to continue taking these products, please check with your healthcare provider to see if there is another option that may be better for you.

Tip

Check the product's expiration date before taking it. By law, all OTC products must have an expiration date. Do not take medicines that have passed this date.

Behind-the-counter medications

Medicines that are kept behind the drugstore counter are technically OTC products because you don't need a prescription to buy them. But, they are kept behind the counter so a pharmacist can speak to you, to make sure that you understand how the drug is used and who should be taking it. Other products are kept behind the counter to control how much of the medication is bought at one time.

Examples of behind-the-counter medications include emergency birth control, and in the U.S., pseudoephedrine, which is found in many products for cold and flu symptoms. In Canada, when pseudoephedrine is sold as a single ingredient, as with Sudafed®, it is also kept behind-the-counter.

Prescription medicines

Prescription medications are drugs that are only available if a healthcare provider has written a specific order for them. There are several types of medicines that could be prescribed for a patient - here are a few of the most common ones:

- Antibiotics - to treat infections. Antibiotics work by preventing bacteria from growing or by killing them. Antibiotics can only treat bacterial infections, not viruses (viral infections), such as colds or the flu.
- Antihypertensives - to treat high blood

pressure. Antihypertensives may be taken alone or with a *diuretic*.

- Diuretics - "water pills" are often used to help treat high blood pressure. These drugs cause your body to remove fluid from your system by making you urinate more often. Diuretics can also cause your body to lose potassium, so be sure to discuss this with your pharmacist.
- Analgesics with opioids (narcotics) - pain killers, to help treat or manage pain. Opioids can be misused, causing addiction, so they are a restricted class of drugs.
- Anti-inflammatories - pain relievers that are stronger versions of the drugs you can buy OTC. Anti-inflammatories help manage pain and other discomfort by reducing inflammation (swelling) in the body.
- Thyroid medication - to treat hypothyroidism. Given to people with underactive or no thyroid.
- Anti-diabetic medications - pills that treat type 2 diabetes.
- Insulin - injectable medicine to manage diabetes, usually type 1, but also taken by some people with type 2 diabetes.

- Cholesterol-lowering medications - to lower low-density lipoprotein (LDL) cholesterol, the so-called "bad" cholesterol.

There are many more types of medication classes and there are usually many varieties in each class. Because there are so many drugs on the market, doctors, nurses, dentists, pharmacists, patients, and caregivers all must be very careful to understand the names of each drug they give or take. Many medicines have names that sound very similar, but they are from different classes. For example:

- *Celebrex* is a drug in the nonsteroidal anti-inflammatory (NSAID) class, and is given for pain. *Celexa* is an antidepressant.
- *Adderall* is a drug made up of amphetamine and dextroamphetamine, which is often given to manage attention deficit hyperactivity disorder (ADHD). *Inderal* is an antihypertensive, for high blood pressure.
- *Amiodarone* is a drug that helps bring an irregular heartbeat to normal. *Amantadine* treats Parkinson's disease.

Vaccines

Vaccines are a type of medicine that is usually only given by healthcare professionals. They usually need a prescription.* Depending on the type of vaccine, vaccinations are available by injection, by mouth, or intranasally (through the nose). Some people refer to these as immunizations.

Some vaccines offer protection from a specific illness for the rest of your life. Some vaccines need boosters after a certain number of years. The seasonal influenza (flu) vaccine is formulated differently every year. The flu virus changes every year, the vaccine must change too. In some states and provinces, the flu vaccine may be given by a nurse or pharmacist without a prescription.

A new type of vaccination is now available in the U.S. and Canada - an oral vaccine that can help prevent "traveler's diarrhea," most commonly caused by a bacteria called enterotoxigenic Escherichia coli (ETEC). No prescription is needed.

Supplements and natural products

Supplements and natural products don't go through the same testing processes as OTC and prescription drugs. Many people believe that if a product is called natural, it must be safe. But this is not always the case. If you choose to take a supplement or a natural product, please talk with your pharmacist to be sure that the product will not interact with any medicines you already take. Some natural supplements should not be taken by people with certain conditions. Your pharmacist can help you with this too.

Conclusion

Taking medicines is an everyday event for millions of people. Because it is so common, it can be easy to forget how serious prescription and OTC drugs can be. Understanding how they work and how best to take them is the first step in reducing risks related to taking medications.

Always keep the following in mind when taking medications:

- Never take someone else's prescription medicine.
- Never give your prescription medicine to someone else.
- Don't take drugs after their expiration date.
- Be sure you know the answers to these questions:
    - Why am I taking this drug?
    - How long do I have to take this drug?
    - How often do I take this drug?
    - How do I take this drug?
    - What side effects should I watch for?
    - Is there anything I should avoid doing, taking, or eating while taking

this drug?
- When can I stop taking this drug?

Abbreviation Glossary

Here are some of the most common abbreviations used with prescriptions and medicines:

AC - before meals

PC - after meals

qd - every day

bid - twice a day

tid - three times a day

qid - four times a day

q4h - every four hours

q6h - every six hours

q8h - every eight hours

q12h - every 12 hours

hs - night time

qhs - every night, usually near or at

ABBREVIATION GLOSSARY

bedtime

qam - every morning

qpm - every evening

prn - as needed, whenever needed

PO - by mouth

PR - per rectum

s/c or sq - subcutaneous

IM - intramuscular

liq - liquid

ung - ointment

gtt - drop

g - gram

mg - milligram

oz - ounces

About the author

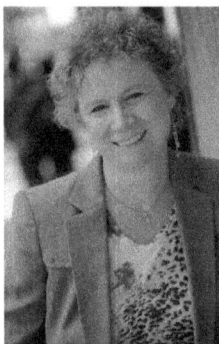

Marijke Vroomen Durning is a Canadian writer
and nurse. Before turning to writing full time,
she worked as an RN in several clinical areas,
caring for both adults and children. She now
works as a health writer and has been
published in outlets including *Costco
Connection*, Forbes.com, *Nursing 2013*, *Alive*,
and more. She has also contributed to
textbooks for nurses and emergency
responders, and she is the author of *Oscar's
Diaries: Life as a Retired Greyhound*.

Thank you again!

Thank you for purchasing *Just the Right Dose: Your Smart Guide to Prescription Drugs & How to Take Them Safely.* I hope you found the information useful and that I answered your questions about prescription drugs.

In order to help spread the word about this book so others can learn about it, I would like to ask you to leave a review of the book either on Amazon) or at the bookstore site from which you bought the book. The reviews help raise the profile of the book so others may find it more easily.

Thank you.

www.ingramcontent.com/pod-product-compliance
Lightning Source LLC
Chambersburg PA
CBHW032153020426
42334CB00016B/1273